The I Am Diet

A Weight Loss Journey of Body, Mind and Spirit

By Sierra Goodman

ISBN 9798586307378

Library of Congress Control Number: 2020924940

THE I AM DIET

A WEIGHT LOSS JOURNEY OF BODY, MIND & SPIRIT

Published in the United States of America

CONTENTS

INTRODUCTION

Welcome to your new happy, healthy life! This book is inspired by my lifetime of yo-yo dieting, my 170-pound weight loss and wanting to share that success with others. Here you will learn how to use the power of your mind to consciously and sub-consciously create the body and life that you desire. I will help you learn how to change your thoughts and emotions to those that will manifest your dreams. You are, after all, a powerful creator with the ability to be, do and have anything you desire, as long as it is for the highest good of all concerned!

Having said that, you must know that when you do reach your goal weight, all your life's issues will not magically resolve. Everyone has had bad things happen in our lives. Everyone has lived through something. But it is up to you if you allow it to empower you or crush you and adversely affect you for the rest of your life. Thin people have problems too. That is why this book will help you to create new thoughts and emotions not only to lose weight, but to also become happy and successful in other areas of your life.

This book is meant to be used as workbook of sorts. I suggest that you read all the way through it and then go through it again, using the ideas and processes to learn how to change your thoughts and emotions to those of a happy, healthy person.

You will find lots of golden nuggets in the Tips, Tricks, Ideas and Inspiration chapter. You can even start there if you want to get a head start on motivation and inspiration.

While physical exercise and specific diets are important, we will be mostly discussing exercising the muscle that is your brain. You are going to learn to think new, healthy, happy thoughts, because it is with flexing our creative muscle called the brain, that we can create a new reality for ourselves. Work that brain, work that brain!

We are going to put our thoughts on a DIET. You are going to learn to think the thoughts that will create what you want, and you are going to learn to let go of and consciously and lovingly change the thoughts that hold you back from your true desires. Conscious focus of your thoughts on what you desire will set you free as you use your power to deliberately create your life. Things will get easier as you follow the inspired ideas and signs that come to you when you focus on your desires.

There are a variety of processes, affirmations, and ideas that I have included here. I encourage you to use your own guidance on which processes you do how often. There is no right or wrong way, only YOUR WAY. Your journey, path, perspective, and preferences are unique to you. Do what feels good to YOU, as that is the first and most important message of this book. After all, I do not want to create "the Sierra Weight Loss Plan," I want you to create your own unique plan that works for YOU with some guidance from me!

You do, however, need to make a commitment to actually do the work. I will make it easier for you as long as you listen to the guided visualizations found on my website, write down and repeat the affirmations and follow the processes. But you have to do it! Make a decision to fight for your life! Stop arguing for your limitations and do the work necessary to become the person you truly want to be!

Nothing is more important than that you feel good. Nothing is more important than that you experience joy and happiness and fulfillment. And it is not up to fate or your past, or others around you that you have given control over your life to for too long. You, right at this moment, can choose the thoughts that will make you happy. All you have is NOW and you get the CHOOSE how you experience your NOW right NOW!

I know all too well what it is like to be judged because of your weight. It is a form of racism. People have already decided that you are lazy and unmotivated. Fat shaming is real and it is something that we have all faced and a difficult burden to bear.

Make the decision that this time you are really going to do it and end the suffering!

You must kick the overeating habit, break your deep emotional ties to food. It has been proven that it takes seventeen days to change a habit. Give me and this book at least that much time. You must be consistent and persistent to break on through to the other side. The happy, healthy side! You are worth it!

I am not a doctor, nutritionist, or any kind of professional that can give medical advice. I am someone who learned how to use conscious and deliberate thinking to attract my desired body to me and I want to share that with you. Please consult your doctor if you feel you need medical advice or before starting any weight loss program. (You know I have to say that!)

I highly recommend listening to my *Becoming Thin Guided Visualizations* while reading this book, as it works to change your subconscious beliefs from fat ones to thin ones, even while you sleep. You will achieve much quicker and easier results. You can purchase them on my website at http://www.iam-iam-iam.com

FIRST THINGS FIRST: WHO YOU REALLY ARE

Before you can start using your deliberate and conscious thoughts to become your healthier, happier, more abundant self, it is important that you truly understand how and why it works. In order to understand why it works, you need to understand who you really are!

You are a physical manifestation of the non-physical super intelligence energy of Love that most people call God. Some people call this Source Energy, Supreme Intelligence, All That Is, Spirit or even The Universe. In this book I use several of those names interchangeably.

Whatever you call our Higher Energy Source or God, YOU are an extension of that. YOU **ARE** THAT! You have a body here in the physical existence, but the larger part of you is your non-physical, higher self; your constant, divine connection to God, who you really are, the I AM that is YOU. Yes, Baby, you are STARDUST on Earth!

Because we are an extension of God in a physical body, we can also co-create our reality by focusing on that which we desire. This is attracting our reality and desires to us with our thoughts. We have this creative ability because we are so loved by All That Is. But we have to do our part of the co-creation. The Universe can more easily give us what we truly want if we clearly ask for it by consciously directing our thoughts to our desires.

We are vibrational beings, and in fact everything that is energy is vibrating. Everything including people, animals, rocks, trees is energy. All energy has a vibration and you attract to you the things that are vibrating at the same wave length as you. We attract things to us that match our vibration, like a magnet.

What you think about, and even more importantly, what you feel and therefore vibrate, you attract to you. If you are feeling bad, you attract more of that feeling to you. If you are feeling joyful and prosperous, you attract more of that to you. You always will get evidence in your life of what you focus on and believe. We are feeling, focusing beings, putting out a vibration depending on how we are feeling, what we are thinking, what our beliefs are, and what we allow into our lives.

This is not about controlling the entire Universe with your mind or thinking that you are better or more powerful than God or the only person in existence. You are a divine spiritual being, a CO-CREATOR with God, who deserves and can have everything you desire and therefore can attract it by using your thoughts and emotions to create what you want. It's a set up that only Divine Supreme Intelligence could have come up with! We get what we focus on by divine Universal Law, which can be explained scientifically with Quantum Physics. I tend to focus on the spiritual side, as for me, science is what explains the divine intelligence of God. Science will always be expanding and learning more about how God put this all together to perfection.

I first learned the Universal Laws in 1986 from an incredible woman named Marilyn Umbach. Marilyn taught me about manifesting the things that I wanted in my life by using the Universal Law of Love. She taught me to write down my goals, dreams, and desires as though I already had them and then use affirmations and other creation tools, like visualization, to put the power in my hands and to trust in the divine order and orchestration of things.

Marilyn taught me that we are the co-creators of our reality and what we think about on a continued basis with passion and emotion, we attract to us. She taught me to not worry about what others were doing, not to push against others, and to only think about what I DO WANT, not what I don't want. If you think about it, even if you don't want it, you bring it into your reality, into your vibrational circle. **That is why we think about and talk about only what we do want, not what we don't want.**

And this is not just about visualizing your life away but *acting* on the Divinely Inspired messages and intuition that will come in magical ways when you create your life in a conscious way and focus on that which you want. And it is about sharing and giving, which in turn, attracts more good to you!

It is YOUR DIVINE RIGHT to have everything you want and so when your vibration matches the vibration of that which you desire, it comes to you by Universal Law as long as it is for the highest good of all concerned. God created this law so that you can have it, but you must do your part and co-create your reality as the powerful Divine Spiritual Being you are! It is your BIRTHRIGHT to have the life of your dreams! Claim it!

Think about it. Where do our desires and dreams come from? Why do we have them? The really great news is that for the most part, what we desire and dream about the things that *are part of our Divine Path and that are ours by Divine Right!* God is not a tease. God is Good. She/He wouldn't have you desire those things if they couldn't be yours! There is nothing you can imagine that you cannot be, do or have, as long as it is for the Good of All and on your Divine Path. Your Divine Path is as incredible as you think your life can be, only better! Your life is only limited by your own thoughts. Start thinking unlimited thoughts! Start to *feel* unlimited!

If you believe that you cannot lose weight, that it is just too hard and that it is your destiny to be overweight, so it shall be. If you believe that you have to work really, really hard to succeed, so it shall be. And if you believe that you are a divine extension of pure Source Energy and that you can have and are worthy and deserving of your desired body, SO IT SHALL BE! It is already true; you just have to embrace it!

We use the Universal Law of Love for weight loss by attracting our desired bodies to us with our thoughts and our inspired actions. In fact, when using this Universal Law, you do not think about fat, or how much you have to lose, or focus on the diets and exercise, you shift your focus to your new body and how you will feel in that new body. We stop thinking about what we have to lose and turn our focus on the new life we will be gaining! You act as if you have it NOW! And when you do that, your guidance and intuition will automatically lead you to the things that will make your becoming thin self-journey easy. You do things that you have been putting off "until I lose weight".

You live your life as if you are already thin, you think thin thoughts like thin people do and then you watch as your body catches up to whom you have already become inside!

It is time to take control of your life, to stop being a victim, to stop blaming others for the things that you feel are wrong in your life and to stop giving over your power to people and circumstances. It is time to become the deliberate conscious creator that you are and create your desires with your deliberate and focused thinking. It is time to tell a new story, give up the one you have been telling, because that old story is holding you right where you are and where you do not want to be.

Your body is listening. Your body is doing just what you are telling it to do. You must find a new way to talk to your body so that there is no resistance to your being thin. If you are sending mixed messages, you will get mixed results.

Tell the story of who you are becoming and what you want, and the Universe will bend over backwards to give you evidence of that in your reality. **Change your perspective, change your life!**

INTRODUCING THE I AM D.I.E.T.

In wanting to inspire others to becoming their thinner self and remember who they really are, I began to think about how to explain the processes I followed to finally release the weight I had been carrying for so many years.

I wanted to find a way to inspire others to really get that YOU are the magic pill you have been looking for to create your desired body and life. I wanted others to know that you define your desires (what you really want) by using your inner guidance. That you give up your resistance to having what you want by identifying your emotions/feelings around worthiness, desirability and food, and then reprogram your thoughts to tell the story of how you want it to be and become it NOW. In this way, it is EASY, easier than taking a pill every day! It is inspiration and connection you are truly seeking, not food. You really need to KNOW and FEEL that you are worthy of being thin and having it all!

I want to guide you to get into a place where it is not a struggle to lose weight, that it is just your way of BEing. When you deal with the emotional and resistance issues around being overweight and around being thin and really *become* the thin person that you want and deserve to be, maintaining a healthy body is easy because it is WHO YOU ARE.

It came to me one day in an instant inspired thought. I could use the word DIET as an acronym and guide for the process because it fit perfectly into what I did! This was a true Divine or Aha! Moment for me because this made it so easy to remember and follow. I felt the excitement and was even more encouraged when I ran it by others, and they were very enthusiastic and supportive of my process.

There is a chapter dedicated to each of these points but here it is in a nutshell:

D –Deservability and Desires: Nothing is more important than that you feel worthy and that you know that you DESERVE all your desires. If you can get this, the rest will easily fall into place. Without feeling worthy of being thin, you would just be struggling on another diet again. After I found my self-worth, or at least was on the road to feeling deservable, I wrote down all my desires around being thin, i.e. I want to wear fashionable clothes, I want to feel good about myself, I wanted to feel healthy, etc. This is where the affirmations really come into play, especially I AM affirmations. After defining my desires, I wrote them in I AM statements, such as I am thin, I am wearing a size 8, I am healthy, I am exercising regularly, etc. Defining your desires creates passion, and passion is a master attractor of your desires!

I – Intuition/Inner Guidance: Learning to use your inner guidance is how you will be led along your journey of self-discovery and becoming thin in the easiest and fastest way possible. I used my intuition and inner guidance to find the right food plan, products and exercises that would serve and work with my body. I listened to my body's guidance on what kinds of food it wanted for nourishment and weight loss. I used my inner guidance and intuition to guide me to the right places, the right people, and to discover my true desires, things that truly inspire me. I asked for inner guidance on what I needed to work on to attract my inner thin person to me, what issues needed work the most.

E - Emotions, Food is tied to emotions, we all have triggers and behaviors and feelings tied to it, whether it is starving kids in Africa, stuffing feelings down, keeping people away, avoiding sex, feeling unworthy, etc. Food is also tied to love for many as our parents gave us food to placate us, and it is even tied to socializing. I identified the emotions I had around food and how I used food to feel better. I then worked my way into new associations with food, little by little, one step at a time. I made food my friend. This is also where self-worth and confidence comes in. I discovered that even though I thought I was a pretty confident person, I was still feeling unworthy of having it all and

I reminded myself that I AM WORTHY!!! I changed my feelings around food to be that which nourishes my body, but not my soul! I can find soul nourishment from within; I don't need food for that.

T - Thoughts, I changed my thoughts about my body, about myself, about food, and replaced these thoughts with new, healthy, high vibing healthy thoughts! This is also where visualization comes in which is a very powerful tool for creation. I started thinking as and BEING the healthy, worthy person that I AM! I found better feeling thoughts, one by one, about food, about my body, and about myself. I used my deliberately focused thoughts to attract my desired body to me.

I knew I had found the perfect name. I am calling my program and book the **I AM D.I.E.T**.! Because that is what I did. I went on an I AM DIET. I AM worthy, I AM thin, I AM, I AM, I AM!

When you say I AM, you are making a statement of who you really are, a self-declaration. It is not I *wish* or I *want,* you are saying I AM. I AM is also another way to say GOD. I AM that I AM implies that the God/Source of the universe is also you. You are part of God. When you say I AM ___, you are acknowledging the God in you. That you are One with God and all that is. That is why I AM statements and affirmations are so powerful!

This should make you think about all those times you have said I AM sick, or I AM bored, or I AM stupid or I AM FAT. It's time to change your I am statements to I AM HEALTHY, I AM JOYFUL, I AM ABUNDANT! Send your I AM statements out to the ethers of the Universe!

This is not a diet as we usually think of diets. This is a LIFETIME PLAN. It is becoming the healthy, trim person you want to be while thinking, feeling and eating like a thin person. It is becoming who you are now, not something you are trying to force or push with pure willpower. It is attracting the thin body that you want to have with your thoughts and feelings. It is attracting what you desire to you by moving molecules and atoms and energy by being a vibrational match to what you want. It is finding your self-worth and self-expression. No regular diet does all that!

So, are you ready to believe that you are special and unique and that you deserve and can have everything you desire and more? Are you ready to acknowledge that you are worthy of all that you desire? Are you really ready to be thin and healthy? Are you ready to give up excuses and blame and all the reasons why you can't and take responsibility and control of your life with your own power of focus? Are you ready to consciously create your life to be everything you want it to be?

I know you have seen other weight loss success stories. I know that you really want that to be you. And it can be, but you need to make the decision that this is it. That this is the time you are going to follow through. You have to really, really want it. You have to BE it. There can be no more next week, next month excuses. There can be no more excuses at all. You are either in or you are out.

If you are not honest with yourself or are not truly ready, this book will just gather dust in a corner of your bookshelf with all the other things that "didn't work for you". These methods will work if you do it and be it *because it is your Divine Right.* You are simply using a Universal Law that is there for all of us to ATTRACT your body and desires to you. But if you don't really, really, really want it, or you don't think you deserve it, it doesn't work.

Unless we have some sort of physical condition or are on medication that creates weight gain, our eating habits and relationships with food are learned behaviors and can be changed and reversed with the desire and motivation and the right tools.

I want to encourage you to find the body weight that is best for YOU. Forget the charts and recommended weights. You will know when you are at the ideal weight for YOU. That might be a bit heavier or lighter than the charts say. Listen to YOU and your body. Every body is different. Bask in your uniqueness!

This is really important: Make peace with where you are. Love all of you, the overweight part of you, love eating, love not eating, love the emotional you, love the procrastinating you, all of you. Let go of your negative self-talk. Go easy on yourself. You are uniquely you! You are not supposed to be like other people. You are on your unique journey as an extension of All that Is, contributing your part to the expansion of thought.

We are going to concentrate on body size of course, but as you are becoming healthier, you can work on the other issues that come up as you become more of who you really are. This is a process, not something that will happen overnight. You can think of it as a butterfly emerging from its cocoon, and it is best to relax and allow yourself to set your own pace along your journey. You cannot rush a butterfly. This is all about unique YOU!

The first thing I recommend before getting started is a really good cleaning of your physical space. This might be your office, or your home, your bedroom, your car or all of these. Cleaning out your space is a great way to feel new and fresh and create room for new things to come to you. Get rid of things that you don't need any more and make room for the new things you will create with your new thoughts. With your space now clean, let us start cleaning up your mind and body!! Let us lighten up in all areas!

D = DESERVABILITY AND DESIRES

Before we start defining your true desires, you must feel deserving and worthy of having them. This will open you up to discovering what it is you really want. After all, you will desire more and manifest it faster if you feel that you deserve it!

You will need a journal or a notebook for this part of your journey. I started off with wire bound notebooks, but I now use smaller journals that I can carry around with me. You should use what works and feels best for you. Just be sure that you have lots of space to write and create! You can also purchase the *I AM DIET Journal* from our website that you can print out and use.

Let us get started with some self-love. On the first page of your journal, make a list of everything that you appreciate about yourself. Everything! As you write, really FEEL the appreciation you have of yourself. Really FEEL how thankful you are that you are YOU! Find all the little things, and the big things, that are wonderful about you!

List EVERYTHING you are appreciative of as this gets you into the appreciative state of mind that is essential for manifesting your desires. Come on, there are so many things that you already love about yourself, about your life! You can do it! Don't be embarrassed or feel that you are being conceited. There is nothing more powerful for manifesting your desires than appreciating and loving YOU!

My friend Osho Rewa, from India, is one of the best rampagers of self-love and worthiness that I know. Here are some lists he has made about what he loves and appreciates about himself. I want to show you how detailed and focused on what you appreciate about YOU that you can and should get. Sit back and read a Master Appreciator!

What are the qualities I appreciate about myself?

- ❖ I appreciate my attention to detail - I notice small things, a slight change in flavor, how the little leaves seem to dance harder during the winds
- ❖ I appreciate how I delight in everyday things like breathing - I really enjoy breathing, once I start paying attention it's like wowza sexy
- ❖ I appreciate my communication skills - I've got an involving, smooth flowing, clear way of writing
- ❖ I appreciate how I intuitively sense people's needs
- ❖ I appreciate that I am passionate about food, I enjoy food so much. I like how I smell food, feel myself touching the food, look at foods closely, yeah totally enjoy food.

- ❖ I like how relaxed about life I am, I know that my life will turn out magnificently. And it is.
- ❖ I like how full of energy I am all through the day.
- ❖ I am a natural inspirer, so many people tell me they find me uplifting, 'a delightful breath of fresh air'
- ❖ I appreciate how honest I am in communicating with people - if I feel it I say it, and I am very very open these days - I feel intimate with everybody
- ❖ I love what an appreciative being I am, and I am so happy that I turned my attention to me now
- ❖ I like how I take care of my body - giving it oil massages, stretching my limbs, eating what I am inspired to, walking, jumping yeah, and I appreciate the acceptance and appreciation I feel for all parts of my body - its heart warming
- ❖ I like that I like myself - what a guy I must be!
- ❖ I like my sense of humor - its free flowing, and I really crack myself up often
- ❖ I appreciate my resonant voice - it's awesome, I can really raise my voice high without shouting, and there's a soothing quality to my voice too –
- ❖ I appreciate how much I delight in my senses - like this morning I woke up to sunlight reflecting off the green trees around, such a sight to see first thing in the morning.

- ❖ I've got a powerful, full smile
- ❖ I like how I care for aesthetics and always look for how to leave things beautifully
- ❖ I like how bold I am, if there's something I want to say, I say it
- ❖ if there's something I really want to do, I do it even if conditions seem adverse
- ❖ I appreciate my frankness - I am a very transparent person
- ❖ I appreciate the enthusiasm I bring to everything I do
- ❖ I appreciate that I delight in the successes of other people; I get so delighted when I hear of people succeeding that I pump my fist! I want to have happy, successful people all around me
- ❖ I like that I am aware of my emotions
- ❖ I love that I have got big desires and I'm passionate about my desires.
- ❖ I appreciate knowing that I am more than my feelings, that I can let my feelings flow through and remain centered.
- ❖ I like that I am confident about myself
- ❖ I enjoy such a deep connection with nature
- ❖ I like that I do what feels best to me

- ❖ I appreciate that I am accepting of myself in all circumstances
- ❖ I like that I am now accepting of other people too in all their diversity
- ❖ I like that I am relaxed and know I don't have to figure it all out
- ❖ I appreciate that I am open to more
- ❖ I like that I dance so totally
- ❖ I like that I'm sport for adventures
- ❖ I like that I like to keep things simple
- ❖ I like that I am straight forward - I speak and act from my heart
- ❖ I appreciate that I feel happy for no reason at all
- ❖ I appreciate that I feel centered all through the day
- ❖ I appreciate that I allow myself as much rest as I require
- ❖ I appreciate that I have attracted peace unto me.
- ❖ I appreciate that I put my feeling good first
- ❖ I appreciate that I am one who is committed to my truth
- ❖ I like myself
- ❖ I am worthy of appreciation
- ❖ I say yes to myself
- ❖ I like that I allow my imagination to flourish
- ❖ I appreciate how fast I can type these days

- ❖ I appreciate that I did the "I love you" mirror exercise today
- ❖ I appreciate that I am open minded
- ❖ I appreciate that I am willing to believe that my life can get better
- ❖ I appreciate that I am not afraid of mistakes or disappointment, why I enjoy them
- ❖ I like that I am working on moving my Self-worth up the emotional scale
- ❖ I appreciate my ability to cook
- ❖ I appreciate my ability to play various sports
- ❖ I appreciate my ability to goof off
- ❖ I appreciate how easily I laugh, how playful I am, how easy going I am
- ❖ I appreciate that I am always looking at the bright side of things

So now you have seen a great example of how to write down and express what you love and appreciate about yourself. While you do not have to do ALL the processes in this workbook, do not skip this one as it is the basis of creating your desires. You have to love YOU! You have to feel deserving and worthy of being at a healthy weight and having your other life desires. So go for it right now! Write all about wonderful, deserving you!

YES, RIGHT NOW!!!!

Another very powerful way to start to feel your self-worth and deservability is to tell yourself how worthy you are while looking in the mirror! Look into the mirror each morning and evening and say I AM WORTHY! I AM WORTHY! I AM WORTHY!!!! I even have a friend that writes this onto her mirror with erasable ink or lipstick. I love this idea!

See, we all need daily reminders, tell yourself EVERY SINGLE DAY that you are Worthy! Do whatever you need to do to start to feel like the WORTHY and DESERVING being that YOU are!!

"You yourself, as much as anybody in the entire Universe, deserve your love & affection."

─ Buddha

The above exercise is never over. You can always add things that you love about yourself every day! Add them in your journal as you think of them.

Now that you are on the road to feeling worthy and knowing who you really are, let's get clear on your true desires around weight loss.

Sometimes to find out what we desire, it is easier to first think about what we don't want. Decide what it is that you are not willing to settle for anymore. Are your knees hurting you? Are you tired of being tired? Are you done with not being able to keep up with your kids? The thing is to think about these things that you don't want and are not willing to settle for, and then change those "NOT thoughts" to what you *do* want. Here is an example of defining your desires from a list of don't wants:

- I don't want my knees to hurt anymore – *I have healthy, strong knees and a bounce in my step*
- I am tired of being tired – *I am full of energy*
- I hate my body – *I love my body as it is now and look forward to how it will be*
- I hate exercise – *I exercise because it feels good and I give myself what I need for good health*
- I do not want my kids to outrun me and tire me out – *I enthusiastically keep up with the kids*
- I don't want my clothes to pull and cut into me – *My clothes fit me perfectly and comfortably*
- I am embarrassed to walk into a room and have people look at me – *I go proudly and confidently wherever I want to go and don't care what anyone else thinks anyway!*

You get the idea. So your final list, after you have changed what you do not want into what you do want, it might look something like this:

My Weight and Body Desires:

- ❖ I am at the appropriate weight for my body type
- ❖ I am a size __
- ❖ I buy any clothes I want, and they fit me comfortably and beautifully!
- ❖ I have energy for all the things I want to do and more
- ❖ I love my body right now
- ❖ I exercise regularly and it feels good
- ❖ I am confident and secure in who I am
- ❖ I am healthy and beautiful
- ❖ I eat appropriate portions and know what foods are good for me and what my body is wanting

It is much more powerful to write things down as if you already have them/are them instead of using "I want" or "I will." However, if that is just too far a stretch for you, if you just cannot yet believe statements such as "I am thin," it is better to at least write down what it is you desire, even if it is still a "I want" and not quite ready to be an "I am". Go easy on yourself. Do what works for you and allow yourself to ease into the new, powerful you that creates their reality!

Another especially important factor in manifesting your desires is to let go of how your wishes and desires will come to you and stop worrying about the how and when of their delivery.

Get out of the way and let the Universe work its magic. Become resistance free and ALLOW YOUR DESIRES TO FLOW TO YOU!

We can get caught up in the how's and when's and actually hold our desires away from us. Once we have clear focus on what we want, we do not focus on the lack of it, we feel it as though we already have it, and then we let go and allow the inspired messages and guidance to come to us.

<u>Affirmations</u>

- ❖ I am filled with light, love and peace.
- ❖ I treat myself with kindness and respect.
- ❖ I don't have to be perfect; I just have to be me, which is perfect!
- ❖ I give myself permission to shine.
- ❖ I honor the best parts of myself and share them with others.
- ❖ I give myself permission to be greater than my fears.
- ❖ I love myself no matter what.
- ❖ I am my own best friend and cheerleader.
- ❖ Thank you for the qualities, traits and talents that make me so unique.
- ❖ I love my body fully, deeply and joyfully.
- ❖ My body has its own wisdom and I trust that wisdom completely.
- ❖ My body is simply a projection of my beliefs about myself.
- ❖ I am growing more beautiful and luminous day by day.
- ❖ I see the divine perfection in every cell of my body.
- ❖ As I love myself, I allow others to love me too.
- ❖ I honor my beauty, my strength and my uniqueness.
- ❖ I love the way I feel when I take good care of myself.
- ❖ My own well-being is my top priority.

I = INNER GUIDANCE & INSPIRATION

We all know or have heard about our intuition or inner guidance. Some call it your soul, or higher being or inner being or higher self or even our sixth sense. I will probably use all of these terms interchangeably because for me, they all mean the same thing: the divine intelligence that is the bigger part of us, the nonphysical part of us that is always connected to divine, supreme, higher, God Source energy. It is who we really are. That inner voice, the intuition, that is the God in YOU.

The non-physical bigger part of you is your inner being and your connection to God source energy. You always have access to that; you always have connection to the divine intelligence within you. We cannot ask for better inner guidance than that!

We *all* have that constant, steady, always ready connection to divine God Source intelligence. You are not the lone human on the planet without this guidance. And people, please, God did not stop talking when the Ten Commandments were handed down to Moses. God still speaks through us, through the voice and guidance of our inner being. How cool is that?

We must learn to hear and trust that inner guidance. We have to trust that there is a higher, divine power at work here through us. We must learn, little by little, to be more like our higher self, who we really are. That is what spiritual growth is, expansion into who we really are, the higher part of YOU.

Your higher self always feels good. That is your natural state. And when you are not feeling good, it is because you are not looking at something from the point of view of who you REALLY are, you are not looking at the BIG picture.

Being your higher self is connecting with who you really are; that thin, healthy, happy person who allows themselves to receive all the good that is theirs by divine birthright. Your higher self knows you are worthy and deserving of all that YOU desire.

Using your inner guidance and intuition is essential for weight loss. You will use this inner guidance to monitor and change your emotions and thoughts, and to choose foods, plans, exercise programs and more. But most importantly, you use your inner guidance to find your inspiration, what turns you on, what makes you go "Oh Yeah, Baby!"

When you are inspired, you are following our inner guidance. When you feel good, you seeing things through the perspective of your higher self. When you are connected with

YOU is when inspired ideas and magical messages and divine signs come easily and frequently. To be inspired is to be in-spirit. When we feel inspired, we are connected to God Source, and from that place we can create anything, including our desired weight.

Overeating is overcompensation for something else you are craving, and that is connection to Source, connection to YOU. ***You are really wanting to feed your soul, not your body.*** That is because on a deep level, you know there is so much more!

Part of being overweight can be that you are not listening to your body and you are not listening to your inner being. It is time to connect yourself with your body by listening to your inner guidance that knows what your body wants and needs. Your body will talk to you in various ways and direct you.

Use your inner guidance to find what inspires you, your true journey or what I like to call my Divine Path. I know that when I follow the divine signs and messages that come to me, when I follow my inspiration, things easily flow into place. Connections, people, places, things come to me that I never could have imagined. That is when I know I am aligned with who I really am.

That is how I knew I was totally aligned with losing weight this time. The journey was easy for me because I had used my inner guidance to show me the way to the right diet, exercise, thoughts and feelings for weight loss.

One thing I have always been pretty good at doing is trusting my guidance. For the most part, I do not care about what others say. But what is funny about me is that sometimes I care more about what people think about the little things, how I am dressed, etc. but when it comes to the big stuff, where I live, what I do with my life, well, no one can tell me what to do!

Who could possibly know what feels good to you, what is good for you, and where you are being divinely led by your divine higher self? Only you!

Only you know what is best for you, you have your own inner guidance, and no one can tell you what that is. You only need to learn to trust it, but really, really trust it. You will use this inner guidance to feel your way to the foods and exercise that will work best for you.

For instance, when I began my weight loss journey, I was called to order and drink Japanese Green tea. Not the Lipton variety, mind you, but the real stuff from Japan. And it wasn't just the constant spam about weight loss with green tea that I kept receiving. I just KNEW it was for me. I felt like my body was calling for it. Every time I saw something about Japanese green tea, I felt something resonate within me. Of course, it turned out to be the closest thing to a magic pill outside myself that I could have found. And I found it by using my intuition, what felt really good to me, not just by reading studies and believing other people's stories of success.

Am I telling you to drink green tea? No, not at all. I am telling you that it worked for me and my body. It might or might not work for you. What does YOUR body say about it? How do YOU feel when you think about it? Does it call to you? Does it make you go "yuck" or "yay?" Listen to that!

Here is another thing I discovered when I really listened to my body and inner guidance. Six smaller meals, instead of three bigger ones, really worked for me. I was never hungry; it was easier and this kept my metabolism up too. Where did three meals per day rule start anyway? Who made that rule? Yes, it is the society norm but does this work for everyone? It does not work for me and I no longer eat that way except when work or other factors dictate that I do. This might or might not work for you. And it is totally okay if it doesn't! This is about YOU and YOUR body!

It is good to have your own beliefs. As you take in lots of information from well-meaning friends, the internet and books, glean what feels good and resonates with you. But it is also important not to get stuck in your beliefs. Keep exploring and expanding what feels good to you as you change and grow spiritually. You are unique and so the exact combination of foods, supplements and exercise is also uniquely yours. You are looking for the choices that feel good to you, what resonates with you, what makes you feel good.

Do not let people convince you that something is good for you and you have to try it because it works for them or they think you should do it. Just because something works for one person, it might not work for another. If you have doubts, there is a reason. Do not let others influence you to do something you do not feel good about. FEEL your way through, listen to your inner guidance and you will be led down the divine path that is right for you! However, if something someone tells you feels good, then do it, because often our guidance comes through others. As you listen to your feelings, your guidance, your heart, you will know when it is meant for you!

"Following another's path leads to who they are,
not to who you are."

— Harry Palmer

The same thing goes for your exercise program. Personally, I suffered through the exercise programs and found that if I feel forced and that I "have to" do it, I will eventually, usually sooner than later, stop doing it. What I found worked for me, was a good walk for cardiovascular exercise and then I did my weight training in small spurts.

I would get up from my computer and do five minutes on my arms. Then a little later I would do a few minutes on my legs, and I would continue this all through the day. When all was said and done, I probably work out more time if I put it all together than I would if I took a twenty minute concentrated time to do it, and the results were the same or better.

Create your own program that works for you and that you will follow. Let it flow with your work schedule, your lifestyle. There are no excuses of "no time to exercise" because you can always find something that will work for you in the time that you have.

Use your own inner guidance on ideas and concepts presented to you. Your guidance is there to lead you on your Path in a divinely guided way, to make it easy and flowing for you. You will just know what resonates with you and will work best for you. Trust it. Go with it. YOU know what is best for you!

If you do not already feel you have a strong connection with your inner guidance, well, you do! You just do not realize it yet. We ALL have that connection; it is just different for each person.

The easiest way to follow your inner guidance is to allow your emotions to be your guide.

Many people meditate to connect more profoundly with their inner being. Some find that guidance can flow out through them by writing or typing in a meditative state, others just ask and hear the answer come into their mind or they are shown in a short time the answer to their question by divine signs and messages. You do not need to sit in the lotus position for hours every day. A short fifteen minutes done consistently each day is all you need to start connecting on a deeper level.

How you communicate with your inner being is very personal to you. And how your higher self-communicates with you is also very unique. Some people feel that their inner being is a female, some a male, some a group of beings. Some people see visions, some hear their guidance like a voice, and for some it is strong urges and impulses... or all of them. There is no right way to connect and communicate with your higher being and your intuition.

Edgar Cayce promoted 'creative writing.' He described this as sitting quietly and in a reflective state, even a spiritually attuned state, and then letting thoughts and ideas flow to you, writing them down as they come. Don't think of these as being for others or for publication. The guidance is for you; it is communication from your higher self, even from God, to yourself.

Sometimes it is a matter of just initiating a conversation with your inner guidance. It could go like this:

"Hi Inner Guidance and Intuition! I would like some guidance about the best weight loss plan for me. Please show me the highest and best answer. Thank you, thank you, thank you!" Then close your eyes and put your consciousness into your heart. If nothing comes right away, do not worry or think that you are doing it wrong. Just let it go and let the divine answer(s) come to you in the right time, in the way that you will receive it and understand it. It might be a news or commentary article that comes to your attention. It might be a street sign or billboard. I've even received Divine Messages from spam email!

You must learn to trust what you receive. It is usually, but not always, the first thing that comes to you. Be open for your Divine Messages to not be what you think it might be. It is essential to get your critical and untrusting mind out of the way and let the Divine shine through!

<u>AFFIRMATIONS</u>

- ❖ I awaken to my higher wisdom.
- ❖ My inner voice guides me in every moment.
- ❖ I am centered, calm and clear.
- ❖ I always know the right actions to achieve my goals.
- ❖ Today I am completely tuned in to my inner wisdom.
- ❖ Thank you for showing me the way to my dreams.
- ❖ I trust my feelings and insights.
- ❖ I am detached and open to divine guidance.
- ❖ The better I know myself, the clearer my purpose becomes.
- ❖ My unique skills and talents can make a profound difference in the world.
- ❖ I follow my heart and discover my destiny.
- ❖ I need not know the entire journey in order to take one step.
- ❖ All is well, right here, right now.
- ❖ Today I embrace simplicity, peace and solace.
- ❖ I trust the universe to deliver my highest good in every situation.
- ❖ I am filled with the light of love, peace, and joy.
- ❖ My inner guidance leads me to the right healing modalities for me.
- ❖ Abundant health and wellness are my birthright.
- ❖ I love taking good care of myself.

E = EMOTIONS

We know that emotions play a HUGE part in eating. We all know about emotional eating and finding comfort through food. We are tethered to long standing chains connecting food to emotions, many of which we are not even aware of, but they are as strong as steel. We can break those chains that bind us by changing our emotional reaction to food. We should eat to nourish our bodies and because it brings us joy. Eating for emotional support or to give ourselves protection and safety is what we are going shift to a new perspective.

Many of our mothers have said, "Eat something, you'll feel better," so when we don't feel okay, food is one of the first things we turn to. Or how about the guilt inducing "Finish your plate, there are starving children in Africa!" We also use food to rejoice and celebrate. Who ever heard of a party without food? We have all experienced that even the smell of certain foods can be an emotional trigger. The mere mention of a dish you remember from childhood can bring up emotions and feelings from years ago. It can feel impossible to separate food from emotions. Food related emotional triggers have earned a prominent spot in your psyche.

Except in necessary situations, most of us do not need years of psychotherapy to let go of the programming and ways of thinking about food that have caused us to gain weight. Do not get me wrong, individual psychotherapy and/or group psychotherapy can be valuable to gain insights and self-understanding on many levels. But there really is such a thing as an "Aha Moment" when a realization can change your life. A new way of looking at something or a new interpretation can allow you to release a belief that has held you back in the past.

If you really deal with your emotions on your current situation, you are cleaning it up in the past too and do not have to go back to that time emotionally to release it. You do not have to go through years of processes and therapies. You can let it go when you recognize it, acknowledge it and are ready.

For example, let us say you were bullied as a child. Based on that experience you decided that you were wimpy, weak, fragile, and pathetic and that is the way you have lived your life up until now. The next time something comes up in your life where you feel that way again, allow yourself to truly and deeply feel the emotion that comes up and then find better feeling thoughts about it, little by little, at your own pace, until you have raised your vibration and feel good about it. You don't have to go back and revisit the embarrassment and pain of the past. You are now officially a conscious creator who can change the way you feel by finding better feeling thoughts in the now moment, from who you have become now. It gets easier and easier as you consciously practice finding better feeling emotions.

You must make a conscious decision to leave the past in the past and move forward with a new future and new ways of thinking and feeling. It is not that hard if your desires are passionate and enthusiastic. You do not need to suffer and dig and go through all the hurt and pain of events and perceptions from your past or do intense introspection to release it. You can decide that it is no longer beneficial for you and let it go! All of the old emotions and fears and blame don't serve you; they are actually harming you, and it is time to move on and be all that you can be! *You deserve it!*

By letting past hurts and pain go, you are *not* saying that what happened is okay. You are not saying that the person who abused you physically or mentally was right. You are just taking away their power to affect *your* life anymore! The situation that left you feeling like a failure that caused you to form negative decisions about yourself can now play out in a different way in your mind. It's your story, you can write it however you want!

Start Telling a New Story!

What story about your life do you tell yourself and others? When someone asks how you are doing, do you go into a tale of how your husband does not treat you well, or how you got screwed in the divorce, that your kids are losers, that you have this illness and that pain, that you can't seem to do anything right, that you'll never be thin, that you are broke, or some other sad story?

The story that you focus on and tell on a consistent basis is what you are creating more of in your life. We get what we focus on. Every time. By speaking constantly of the things we don't want, we create more of it in our lives. We speak of it to anyone who will listen, we join groups about it, we tweet about it, we blog about it, and there it is. Always. We just keep getting more of what we do not want, created by ourselves by focusing on the things we don't want and holding them close to us.

But what if we start to tell the story how we want it? What if when someone asks how we are, we focus on all the GOOD in our lives. What if we start creating a new story? A great example of this is a woman who wrote to me with a long, sad story detailing what she wanted to do, but all the reasons why she couldn't do them. She was limiting herself and holding herself back with her own words. This is what I wrote to her:

Now take a few minutes and write the story the way you want it to be, with the outcome that you want. If your heart is in the writing of the story the way you want it to be, then you will feel the shift of energy for that to actually begin to manifest. Remember, you can be do and have anything you want. Continue only to write and tell the story the way you want it to be and this creates the passionate and positive energy flow to make all of it come to pass quickly and easily.

I cried tears of joy when she wrote back to me:

Thank you for your email - you are right. I have re-read your email a few times and I do agree...I have re-written my story. I carry it with me everywhere I go and I look at it when I feel slightly down. I thought I would share it with you:

"I am a beautiful woman with exotic features and a gorgeous body. I am at my perfect weight all the time. I love my body and feed it well - I follow whatever my palette desires, food is indeed my friend. I love my work-outs and dressing up in the morning - this is my time to re-connect with myself and revel in the joy of being ME. Life is very natural and easy for me, I receive ABUNDANCE in all areas of my life - health, wealth, professionally and in all my relationships. All opportunities are presented to me in good time, in alignment with my vibrational offering. I believe that all is vibration and I believe in miracles. I thoroughly enjoy what I do for a living. I believe strongly that personal power comes in pursuit of one's passion. I believe I can have it all - and I know it will come easily to me. As I begin to become clear about my career and its path, I will begin to see progress, change and success. I am surrounded my endless opportunities for success and I am not limited by my current place of residence. There are many like me who have desired their jobs into being and I can do the same. I am an inspiration to myself first and I am bound for success!"

This is how to tell a new story! Stop talking about the things that you do not like and want to let go of. Start talking about the things that you want to come to pass as if you have them right now. Practice telling your new story as often as you can. It might take you a while to stop telling your old one since you have been telling it for so long. But you will soon see that you stop yourself when the old story begins to come out and instead you tell your new one. And then it will become automatic and you will be amazed how quickly your new story becomes reality. The faster you become it, the faster it becomes you!

One of the things that I discovered about myself is that I used food to stuff my feelings. Although I can be very long-winded in my writing, I am often quiet in front of people. I was afraid to say what was on my mind or what I was feeling and instead, I would stuff my feelings down with food. I was afraid that people would think of me in an unfavorable way if they really got to know me so if I kept quiet, they would not be able to judge me. Through self-discovery, I have learned to feel better about myself and I am now longer fearful of people getting to know me. Further, and even more profound, is that I now know that what others think about me is not as important as what *I* think of me.

When I started paying attention to my thoughts and emotions, I noticed that eating and procrastinating had a big connection for me. Whenever I had a project that I did not want to work on, I would find myself thinking about food. I used food as a distraction. When I find myself overeating, I stop and ask, "What is it I am not saying?" "What is it I am not doing?" "What is it that I am using food as an excuse to not deal with?"

I have lost weight before. Many times. My weight loss never lasted for very long until I was able to understand my resistance to actually staying thin after I got there. It was a scary world that I had not properly allowed myself to prepare for emotionally. I had to give up my fear of having it all (feeling worthy), my fear of speaking my mind (not afraid of judgment) and my fear of not having any more excuses to not be all I could be.

I could use willpower and motivation to lose weight, but I would always gain it back plus more because I had not really gotten in touch with the true reasons why I was overweight. Be honest with yourself about all of your excuses and reasons. You do not need them anymore! You are entitled to be the best you can be! You deserve it! You can begin to create your new dream life right now, today, this very **minute!**

WHEN YOU BEGIN TO OVEREAT, ASK YOURSELF, "WHAT'S EATING AT YOU?"

I ate because I was bored, stressed, depressed, upset, too busy, or because it was raining. I was substituting chocolate for conversation, pasta for a full bank account and bread for being happy. It didn't need to be a major disappointment or a life changing event for me to seek solace from food. I was doing what I had always done. Changing those triggers to healthy choices took me making a U-turn in my thinking!

Most of us cannot go from sad to happy in a heartbeat and in fact, by doing that, we can sometimes be avoiding the issue instead of consciously raising our vibration and feelings about it. But you can go from sad to hopeful by consciously changing your perspective, step by step, one emotion at a time, at your own pace.

You will get better and better at raising your vibration, at changing your thoughts on any issue as you practice and let go of your resistance. The more you resist an emotion or situation, the more it persists. Just try pushing that anger away without feeling it first. It just builds up. It persists. Feel it, then let yourself move on to the next emotion that feels better than anger.

I had to learn to recognize true hunger. Often hunger and cravings can be a disguise for actually craving human contact, a conversation or a fulfilling and healthy life.

If I was not going to use food for comfort, I had to find some good substitutes. Sometimes I needed to leave the scene of temptation, to go for a walk or to take a shower. Often, calling a friend or getting into some other enjoyable activity would be the key. Whatever I needed to do to postpone eating when I *knew* it wasn't about hunger was the new response. I kept myself busy and changed my thoughts to the thoughts of a thin person. It is a process. Go easy on yourself. Stay deliberately and consciously focused on your goal.

I now know that in every moment I have a choice of what to think about and a choice of how to feel. That makes me boss of my world! I am in charge of me! How exhilarating is that?

The goal is to start becoming aware of the things you have been doing as a *reaction* rather than a *decision*. Repetition and practice is the best thing you can do to change a lifelong response. It is possible! It can take a long time to change ALL your resistance and beliefs but pick and choose the ones to work on NOW.

The following process allows you to plan the future so that next time you are ready to reach for food, you have an alternative ready without thinking about it too much.

List 10 things that you could do when the refrigerator is calling you. Choose things that you enjoy: Here's a few of mine to get you going:

- ❖ Take a walk
- ❖ Work in the garden
- ❖ Write/answer emails
- ❖ Call a friend
- ❖ Take a bath
- ❖ Dance to great music
- ❖ Appreciate my surroundings
- ❖ Work on a project
- ❖ Pet your dog/cat
- ❖ Internet shop (you don't actually have to buy!)

Keep your notebook with the list you create available so that you have them when you need to refer to them in weaker moments.

I found this next exercise profoundly helpful. I made a list of all the issues I had around being thin - and there are always issues; otherwise, you would already be there. There is something(s) you are gaining by being overweight besides fat. I knew that I had to get to the root of the emotions that triggered overeating so that I could change those emotions to different associations.

Questions to ask yourself to get started:

- ❖ What am I gaining by staying overweight?
- ❖ What does being overweight allow me to do or not do
- ❖ What are your fears around being thin?

It is good to find your resistance in these areas and work on them little by little. Here are some things you may relate to:

- ❖ People wouldn't like me anyway
- ❖ No one can tell me what to do
- ❖ I don't have to compete in fashion
- ❖ I don't have to compete in life
- ❖ I can turn to food when I'm feeling sad/happy
- ❖ I don't have to change my habits
- ❖ I can eat instead of tackling that project
- ❖ I don't want to stir up the past
- ❖ A lot more would be expected of me if I was thinner
- ❖ I don't want people to get too close
- ❖ I don't have to do physical things
- ❖ I don't have to have sex

- ❖ I have an excuse for people not to like me
- ❖ People feel sorry for me
- ❖ It's my Mom/Dad/Brother/Sister/Mate's fault
- ❖ Being fat fits my fat self-image (that's the way I always have been and always will be)
- ❖ I eat "instead of" studying, cleaning, making that call, etc. (procrastinating)
- ❖ I eat to cover up unresolved anger/depression, shove down your feelings
- ❖ I don't have to compete finding love
- ❖ Not as much is expected of me if I stay overweight.
- ❖ I stay fat because no one can tell me what to do (it's one thing that is totally in my control)
- ❖ Being fat is comfortable - I KNOW how to be fat, I don't know what it's like to be thin (fear)
- ❖ I have extremely low self-esteem and feel undeserving
- ❖ I feel that success is for the lucky people but not me
- ❖ I believe that losing weight may require me to make a major life change (i.e., get a divorce, change jobs)
- ❖ I fear that my friends will not like the new, confident me

If you see yourself in any of the above reasons for staying overweight, or you have other reasons of your own, it is time to decide if you are ready to give those up. How does holding on to old hurts, pain, and blame serve you in your life now? How does being overweight serve you? Really think about this. Your present life is serving you in some way or you would not still be overweight/broke/unhappy. What do you gain by being overweight or non-successful? There is definitely some payoff for you, and you need to figure those out so that you can re-wire your thinking so that the payoff is in being thin, not overweight!

It is also time to give up the blame game. Your ex/Mom/Dad/sister/brother/friend are not suffering because you feel bad, *you* are the one who feels bad. By hating or blaming others for how your life is going, you are only attracting more of the same negative feelings back to YOU, not to them. Why give others that power over your life? Let us stop that right now! As a Divine Spiritual Being, you only need to let go of those past feelings and start living the life that you deserve.

Now, here's the fun part! Rip out and crumple up the paper with all your excuses and reasons for staying overweight. Rip it up into a thousand pieces or burn it. Or do all these things! Do whatever makes you feel as you have just released all your old ways of living to open space for a new way of living! Laugh and Release as you rip up all your past stuff and watch it burn. It is fun and you will feel incredibly wonderful and free as you release your old way of being and doing things and instantly transform into the new you!

KNOW YOUR TRIGGERS.

Write down what you eat, how much you eat, when you eat, how you are feeling when you eat and how hungry you are. Be honest, this is just for you. Over time, you will see patterns emerging that can help you notice and change your habits and responses. You may be very surprised to notice that eating is rarely a response to hunger. Make a table in your notebook or journal (or use our I AM DIET Journal)

DATE	WHAT FOOD I AM EATING	HOW MUCH I AM EATING	TIME OF DAY	HOW AM I FEELING BEFORE AND DURING EATING	HUNGER LEVEL AT THE TIME OF EATING

After a few days, take a look at your entries. Look for patterns; is it always salty food? Is it often in the evening and rarely when you're hungry? Is it when you're bored, sad, angry?

Now, this is important. You are observing your triggers for emotional eating. But do not keep the focus on your emotional eating triggers or get down on yourself for doing it. Just observe the pattern, and then pivot your thoughts away from emotional eating when the triggers arise. You observe the behavior you want to change and then shift your focus to the behavior you want to create, not stay stuck in focusing on the behavior you don't want anymore.

Here's another good process that really helped me to enjoy food in a whole new way. I used to inhale my food. I was always the first one done and I was a proud member of the *"CLEAN PLATE CLUB"*. Sometimes I would remember to slow down, but most times not, it was a HABIT! I finally made myself a little card that I put on the table when I ate meals. It said:

- ❖ Stay Present!
- ❖ Think about what you are eating!
- ❖ Slow down, enjoy your meal and CHEW, CHEW, CHEW!
- ❖ Stop eating when you are full!
- ❖ It is okay to leave food on my plate. Worms and bugs need food too, it will get eaten by something eventually, it doesn't have to be me.

I used this card until I did not need it anymore. It was just one of the little games and methods I played with myself while I practiced changing my beliefs, behaviors, resistance, and vibration.

When I find myself eating for emotional reasons, I go through a series of questions to myself:

- ❖ What is it that I am not saying?

- ❖ What am I not letting myself feel?
- ❖ Why am I bored?
- ❖ Am I focused enough?
- ❖ What do I need to seek clarity on?
- ❖ Why am I feeling uninspired?
- ❖ Who do I need to talk to?
- ❖ Am I letting others trigger me?

So, let us get rid of these past thoughts, feelings and associations that no longer serve you. Let us take an honest look at all of the reasons why you are not living the life of your dreams right now as you let your emotions rule your desires.

In your journal or notebook, write down all the excuses you have used for why you are not doing what you want to be doing. Write down everyone you blame for your present situation and why they are stopping you from living your dream life. Write down all the reasons why you are not living the life of your dreams right now. Write down your whole sad story. Think of all the things in your life you have just settled for because you thought you could not do or deserve better. Think of how much you let others control who you are and what you do. Some examples are:

- ❖ I am too busy taking care of the kids to work on me

- My husband/wife/partner will not let me do what I want to do
- It is my parents' fault for the way they raised me
- I blame my wife/husband/teachers/sister/brother for the way my life is
- I am just not that kind of person who can do those things
- It is my boss' fault
- My husband/wife left me and ruined my life
- My teacher/parent/partner doesn't understand me, in fact, no one understands me
- My accident made me this way
- My parents divorced when I was young and it was tragic for me
- I was abused/raped
- The drugs/medications I take make me this way
- I was told I would never amount to anything and I believe it
- I can't do any better than my present boyfriend/girlfriend/husband/wife/partner
- I can't get a better job

Keep going until you feel you have written all the reasons why you are stuck in the situation you are now. Write them ALL down, this is for you and you do not want to cheat yourself.

Remember you want the smorgasbord, not the fast-food version of life! Take your time and really think why you do not do what you want to do in life. What are you allowing to stop you? Who are you allowing to stop you? Who, or what are you using as an excuse to not be all that you can be?

Isn't it time to let that go and take responsibility for your own life, for your own vibration and what you are attracting? Isn't it time to give up the blame game? YES!

So, now take all those statements of blame and injustice and suffering at the hands of others that you just wrote and write out how you now take responsibility. Take your negative statements and make them into positive ones. "It is my parents' fault for the way they raised me." becomes "My parents did the best they could, and it is up to me to control my life now." "I am just not that kind of person who can do those things" becomes "There are unlimited possibilities for me. I am only limited by my own thoughts. I can do things now that I never thought possible before." Write from your knowledge that you are the creator of your reality. Write from knowing that you are deserving and worthy of your desires. Write knowing that as long as you keep telling your old story, you are holding yourself there... so make it good!

Another great exercise to do, especially if you are having trouble getting into the feeling place of being thin is playing "What If." *What if* I was thin? *What if* I could buy all the cute clothes I wanted? *What if* I was with my perfect mate? What If allows you to dream, visualize, and feel it without making statements that you just cannot yet believe or feel. It is a way to get yourself daydreaming and *feeling*.

Another version of this is "Wouldn't it be nice?" *Wouldn't it be nice* if I weigh 140 pounds at my class reunion? *Wouldn't it be nice* if I fit into my college jeans? Let yourself daydream and get into the feeling place. That is how you can slowly change your statements into ones that you truly believe are true and therefore will create. Wouldn't it be nice if I could fit into my college jeans turns into I AM WEARING MY COLLEGE JEANS!!!

<u>Affirmations</u>

- ❖ I am perfectly healthy in body, mind and spirit.
- ❖ I am well, I am whole, and I am strong and healthy.
- ❖ I am healthy, and full of energy and vitality.
- ❖ All the cells of my body are daily bathed in the perfection of my divine being.
- ❖ I am healthy, happy and radiant.
- ❖ My body is a safe and pleasurable place for me to be.
- ❖ My sleep is relaxed and refreshing.
- ❖ I have all the energy I need to accomplish my goals and to fulfill my desires.
- ❖ My body is in balance, restored and filled with energy.
- ❖ I love and accept myself unconditionally.
- ❖ I radiate love and respect and in return I get love and respect.
- ❖ I am a well loved and well respected person.
- ❖ I am a cultured and wise and yet, a humble person.
- ❖ My high self-esteem enables me to respect others and beget respect in turn.
- ❖ I am free to make my own choices and decisions.
- ❖ I am a unique and a very special person and worthy of respect of others.
- ❖ My high self-esteem allows me to accept compliments easily and also freely compliment others.

- ❖ I accept others as they are and don't care what they think about me.
- ❖ It matters little what others say. What matters is how I react and what I believe.
- ❖ All is well in my world and I trade love and acceptance with the world.
- ❖ I have high self-esteem as I respect myself.
- ❖ I deserve all that is good. I release any need for misery and suffering.
- ❖ I release the need to prove myself to anyone as I am my own self and I love it that way.
- ❖ I am never alone. The universe supports me and is with me at every step.
- ❖ My mind is filled only with loving, healthy, positive and prosperous thoughts which ultimately are converted into my life experiences.
- ❖ My mind is full of gratitude for my lovely and wonderful life.
- ❖ I consciously release the past and live only in the present. That way I get to enjoy and experience life to the full.

T = THOUGHTS

Most of you have heard it before. THOUGHTS BECOME THINGS. What you think about continuously, and especially those things you think about with strong emotion, is what you create and attract to you.

What have you been thinking when you look in the mirror? Have you been critical and demeaning of yourself? Have you made your own harsh opinions and judgments about your body the truth by saying it over and over again? You are probably much harder on yourself than you would be on anybody else. It is time to turn that around. Cut yourself some slack and think about what you are doing right. Focus on your good points. Focus on all that is good and stop putting yourself down.

Think about the thoughts that you have made into facts about food such as when you eat, how much you eat, the foods you choose, how much is enough. WHO SAYS SO? You can rewrite those rules anytime you choose to. These rules are only true because *you* say they are.

Right now you can decide to get rid of all your "should haves" and "could haves" and "why didn't I's." You can train yourself to be impeccable in your thinking and use your thoughts to create the life you desire.

Just the phrase, "I think I can" is hopeful and optimistic as opposed to "I can't" or "I could never do that." Use your ability to choose your thoughts to help yourself – not hurt yourself. When you are not happy with yourself, you can forgive yourself and visualize yourself doing it the way you want to. Use your thoughts to leave any situation or circumstance in a positive light.

Train your mind to consciously visualize the things that you want, not the things that you do not want. Thinking about negative things that could or might happen uses up your energy and you are actually attracting those things to you by constantly thinking about them.

If you think about falling and worry about falling, you are increasing the chances of you falling. By thinking about it, you are only putting your energy towards and attracting the thing that you are worried about. Instead, put your thoughts on the best possible outcome of the situation. It is not so hard once you get the hang of it. And you will feel so much better in *all* areas of your life!

I THINK, THEREFORE I AM THIN.

Listen to what you say to yourself. Pay attention to your choice of words. Listen to your self-talk. Listen to the story that you tell about yourself. Do you put yourself down? Do you play the martyr? Pay attention to the thoughts that you think. Wouldn't it be far more helpful to say, "I am becoming leaner and healthier every day" instead of saying, "I have always been fat and I probably always will be?"

When you find your thoughts wandering to non-productive things, just smile and consciously change the thought to something positive. Find a pivot thought, something that automatically makes you happy and use that when you need it.

For instance, when I find myself in a negative state of mind, sometimes I cross my arms and blink my negative thoughts away. I call it the I Dream of Jeannie method. I remember things that make me happy, like hanging out with dolphins and whales, or my animals, or fun times I have had.

It is best to have a predetermined trigger thought or thoughts that you can grab onto quickly if needed. Once you pull yourself out of a negative mind spin, you can go back and clean up your thoughts around the issue, one at a time, replacing your negative thoughts with your new, positive thoughts.

It helps me to play the game of thinking of all the reasons why whatever is bothering me is a good thing, or at least an OK thing. For example, what if I lost my wallet? I could let it start me on a negative spiral that ends up with overeating or, I could remind myself that I just have to make a couple of phone calls to fix it and I needed a new wallet anyway. Maybe the person that gets it didn't have a wallet at all. Maybe they needed the money more than I did.

Instead of letting the circumstance get me going in a negative direction, I work to find reasons why it is ok even if I have to stretch a bit at first. It is a process to work yourself into better and better feeling thoughts, especially about things that trigger strong negative emotions in us.

You can cross your arms, blink your eyes and 'Jeannie' your old thoughts and feelings away. Maybe you relate more with Elizabeth Montgomery in Bewitched. Whether you blink your eyes, wiggle your nose, tap together your Ruby slippers, use the Force, tie a yellow ribbon around the old oak tree, or beam yourself up, the important thing is to just let it go and switch to positive, upbeat, life changing thoughts. The idea is to make this fun and very personal to what works for you. Create your own mind training games with things that you can relate to and will actually use.

It takes practice and patience, and you will get better and better at it every single day! It is so worth the effort. You will have a whole new outlook on life on all levels.

VISUALIZE YOUR SIZE!

I have found visualization to be an extremely powerful tool in the journey to transform my life. Here's one that I've used a lot: Visualize yourself as the thin person you want to be. Close your eyes and feel how it feels to walk like a thin person. Feel the bounce in your step. Feel the feeling of zipping up those smaller jeans without lying on the bed (unless you want them that tight!) Visualize yourself going into your favorite store and buying smaller sizes. Imagine the details, the smells and feelings in vivid living color detail. Visualize yourself walking into a room as your thin self and feel your confidence and joy. Visualize yourself at a healthy weight, full of energy, confidence and optimism. Do this as often as you can – it will become the way it actually is!

You can do these visualizations on your own or check out my *Becoming Thin Guided Visualizations* available on my website.

Denis Waitley, a world famous coach and motivator told Olympic athletes in training to visualize hooking the basket, hitting the home run, crossing the finish line. Make it as real as possible. Begin to walk, talk, think and eat like the thinner person you want to be. Think to yourself, "If I was thinner, how would I walk? Would I walk taller? How would I eat? How would I think? Would I be sitting here on the couch watching soaps or the football game and eating potato chips or would I be out doing something?" Paint the picture in your mind of exactly what your life would be like if you were thinner, and do it, be it! Now!

The ability to always consciously choose your thoughts is not going to happen overnight. It also is not going to happen if you turn it into something that you only do when you notice it on your "do to" list. It must become who you are, how you are and what you are. It takes time and patience.

Start by noticing your "self-talk." Listen to the voices in your head and decide if you want that message or not. If not, gently change your train of thought. If you need to, picture a pink elephant or imagine a scene from a favorite movie – anything that helps you change your track.

Visualization is just another form of using your imagination. Visualization allows you to visualize the best possible outcome. You get to create it in your mind exactly the way you want it.

You can daydream or play house or do whatever you did as a kid when you played in your mind. It is the same thing, but as adults, we forget the wonderful world of our imagination. We forget that our imagination is there to help us create our reality! Imagine your reality as you want it, feel the feelings and passion of it being real and watch the molecules move in your favor! The Universe is conspiring FOR YOU!

Even if you are not ready to believe that you can guide your thoughts, go through the motions. Do it anyway! Fake it until you make it! It certainly won't do you any harm and it just might change your life!

Attitudes and beliefs about food and eating come from our thoughts and programmed behaviors. Some of us have thoughts that we have thought our whole life. Following is a letter from a "thin" person about her beliefs.

"One day I decided to stop looking at food as the enemy and realized it could just as easily be a friend. After I befriended food, I felt free to befriend exercise and found the perfect program that after getting the "work" done, only takes three 15 minute workouts a week to maintain."

It is good to ask your "naturally" thin friends what their attitudes and beliefs are about food. You can then take on some of those beliefs. I have friends who honestly believe that they can eat anything and they will not get fat. And they don't!!

You cannot possibly monitor all the thoughts that you have every day. This is just the beginning of being aware and the more aware you are, the sooner you will feel better about yourself, the people and things around you and life itself. Have fun with this, laugh at yourself and treat yourself well. *Practice makes permanent.*

Make yourself unlearn what you thought was true. Stop making excuses and putting up hurdles to jump through. You must rewire your brain to ease the struggle and truly live with a whole new way of thinking and eating.

By listening to my thoughts, I have learned a lot about myself. I have learned that my weight reflects how I am feeling about myself and my world. I have always used food to stuff it down when I am not saying what I want to say or doing what I want to do. For me, excess weight is a symptom of NOT BEING WHO I REALLY AM, of suffocating myself. That is why the concept of **"I AM"** is so important to me and why it is the name of this book and my website.

After all the weight I have lost, I am determined to not go back there ever again. Now I quickly catch myself when I am using food as an excuse to not be WHO I REALLY AM. It is an on-going process, but now I am able to catch it faster. It really does get easier. With the tools I have learned to use, I am able to work through the reasons I am overeating and get myself back to acting like the thin person I REALLY AM. At the end of this chapter, I have some tools for you to use. I think of them as games I play with myself – and **I AM** always the winner!

Visualize and consciously feel how you want your life to be and do not negate it with doubts and negative thoughts. You can do all the visualizations, journaling and processes in the world and it will not work if you negate all that positive work with negative, doubting thoughts. Trust and have faith! Act as if it was already true and it will be soon!

YOU ARE IN CHARGE OF THE WAY YOU THINK ABOUT THINGS!

My decisions and judgments about things and people are just that – my decisions and judgments. It is my unique perspective. Knowing that, I appreciate and accept others as much as I am working on appreciating and accepting myself. As an example, I worked to appreciate people who were at a healthy weight and not be envious. I was on the way to being lean and strong and I began to look at them as an example, as an inspiration. I applied this credo to other people and things and found myself much more peaceful. Wayne Dyer, the famous author and philosopher said, ***"When you change the way you look at things, the things you look at change."***

There are many processes using visualization. If you have a favorite, use it. The goal is to visualize yourself at your goal weight looking lean and strong and full of health. Make it real, make it vivid, make it detailed. See the clothes you are wearing, know the way they feel, feel the confidence.

My 'visualization place' is on a cliff overlooking the ocean. When I go there, I leave the world behind and am mentally prepared to visualize. I have a closet there with many different outfits in the size I want to be, with accessories to complement them. Anything goes in my 'visualization place' and I can be, do or have anything I choose. I like to think of it as a dress rehearsal! That is what visualizing is – creating your life how you want it to be with your imagination.

Find a quiet place away from interruption or distraction. Turn off the phone and just relax and breathe for a minute. Let your imagination roam with the idea of looking for your 'visualization place'. Find a place that you are comfortable and feel safe. Take your time with this and let it unfold. This is your place, make it the way you want it, decorate it however you'd like. If you find your mind roaming, bring it back. Try to stay with it until you have a clear picture of your place. Be sure to remember every detail so that you can now go back there whenever you choose.

Now this visualization place becomes where you go in your thoughts, whenever you can, whenever you want to explore the thinner, healthier you. In your place, you can try a sport you have always wanted to try, you'll run with ease with your hard lean body. Try on clothes you would love to wear and notice how nice it is to wear clothes that skim your body without being tight. Do the things you have postponed doing in your imagination – and you will be ready when your body catches up with you. Trust me, this is a most powerful part of becoming proud of saying, **I AM**.

If you are having trouble doing visualizations on your own or just want extra help, I highly recommend my Becoming Thing Guided Visualizations found on my website.

Another great tool for conscious creation and speaking subliminally to your sub-conscious are Vision Boards. I love seeing the photos of coming attractions in my life go by and feeling the feelings of already having them NOW. You can also cut and paste photos from magazines and place them around where you can see them.

Deliberately pivoting your negative thoughts to positive ones, visualizing and becoming your thin self in your mind, acting as if you are already there are your magic pills to becoming the thin person you want to be!

<u>Affirmations</u>

- ❖ I experience Love wherever I go.
- ❖ I handle all my experiences with wisdom, with love and with ease.
- ❖ I rejoice in my uniqueness.
- ❖ I deserve to be successful.
- ❖ I move beyond old limitations and now allow myself to express freely and creatively.
- ❖ I care about myself.
- ❖ I deserve good in my life.
- ❖ I am lovable because I exist.
- ❖ I am willing to feel. It is safe for me to express my emotions. I love myself.
- ❖ I feel good about my life.
- ❖ I speak up for myself.
- ❖ I am self-confident.
- ❖ I am in control of my life.
- ❖ I am inspired by life.
- ❖ I am proud of my accomplishments.
- ❖ I am filled with positive energy.
- ❖ I cherish myself.
- ❖ I am safe just being me.
- ❖ I am good enough just as I am.
- ❖ I express my self-confidence and self-worth.
- ❖ I am a good person.
- ❖ I am worth loving.

TIPS, TRICKS, IDEAS & INSPIRATION

Even though this book is about deliberately focusing our thoughts on what we want, I want to share some things that really helped me become happier and healthier because maybe they will help you too! However, do not just do what I did because it worked for me, the key is to find your own unique journey and the tips and tricks that inspire you. I am with you! I support you! GO FOR IT!

I am including here some weight loss and manifestation tips, tricks, ideas and inspiration that I found very helpful for me to get started and keep going. You didn't think you were going to completely get out of the exercise thing did you?

❖ **Get a kick start with a strong motivation.** It can be very useful to find a strong motivation to change your current eating habits and lifestyle to help give you a jump start. For each individual person, "the thing", the one thing that finally motivates you to go for it, is different. You have to find your thing; the person, or place, or photo, or health issue that motivates YOU.

I recommend taking pictures of yourself so you can no longer avoid knowing what you look like to others. You have to be honest with yourself, even if you are not honest about your weight on your driver's license! Sometimes the photos alone are enough to motivate you. If that doesn't do it, maybe there is some hot guy you like (or some husband you want to keep!), or a trip you want to take, or a cute outfit that you want to look good in. Whatever your motivation is, post it on the fridge and all around your house and keep it in the forefront of your mind at all times.

I kept several things in my mind during my weight loss. One was a photo of me looking like the Goodyear Blimp's younger sister. The other was that my knees were starting to go and I pictured myself having to use a lift system to get up the stairs to my house. That one really motivated me!

❖ **Use the power of affirmations.** Saying affirmations is a very powerful message to the universe and to your sub-conscious mind when you write down your hopes and dreams as if you already have them. I used a journal and wrote things like: "I am healthy and thin", "I weigh 130 pounds", "I am a size 8". You get the idea. I use affirmations as needed, but find it best is in the morning before I start my day and right before I go to bed. Remember, affirmations only work if you believe them, so you might start out with "Wouldn't it be nice if..."

until you find the feelings and emotions that create what you are affirming for.

❖ **To go with your written affirmations, VISUALIZE YOURSELF as the thin person you are**. Visualize yourself in the clothes you want to wear, FEEL IT, BE IT! This is an important part of weight loss, do not skip this step, it really helps! One of the things I did is when I was huffing and puffing up the 72 steps to my house was that I pictured myself bouncing and even running up those steps. Now it is true! Visualize yourself on vacation on the beach in a bathing suit, visualize yourself buckling your seat belt without holding in your stomach, visualize yourself zipping up adorable Size 5 jeans with ease. The more you do this, the easier your weight loss will be. Trust me on this.

❖ **It is so important to do things that make you feel good about yourself during this time**. Please take off those ugly sweats, cut them up and use them for cleaning the house and buy yourself some new clothes that you feel good in, no matter what size they are. NO FRUMPS!!!! EBay, and Alight.com were a Godsend for me as I was able to buy really cute plus size clothing that made me feel great. Don't go crazy, because your new clothes won't fit you for long! Keep cleaning out your closet as clothes get too big on you. Donate them or even sell them on eBay. Don't keep around "fat clothes" just in case. You don't want to have that to fall back on. Don't create safety nets for yourself this time. Go for it or Go HOME! Get a manicure, get your hair done, and treat yourself like the princess (or prince) that you are! The trick is to keep you feeling good about yourself and not fall back into self pity and overeating. Shift your focus!

❖ **Raise your hand if you are a member of The Clean Plate Club.** Yep, I thought so. I am the same way, there are starving children in Africa, you know. I have learned to ask for smaller portions because it is so hard for me to leave food on my plate. If you are still served too big portions, repeat after me, "It is okay to leave food on my plate. Worms and bugs need food too, it will get eaten by something eventually, and it doesn't have to be me." Keep saying it. Stop eating when you are full. It is always good to drink a big glass of water ten minutes before you eat. You will feel fuller faster and will have that extra motivation and willpower that you need!

❖ **Find a food plan that works for you and that you can stick to.** What is important is that it is a program that you can stay on without feeling deprived and hungry (feeling deprived leads to overeating!) and that will support you after you have reached your goal. I am constantly changing what I eat. I go through phases of eating one type of a food or another and then switching as I listen to my body's needs. In general, I stick with a plan that I call the **Sierra's Super S Lifestyle** and that is Smoothies, Salads and Soups. Of course sometimes I eat other things, but if I stay with this way of eating on most days, I can keep my weight where I want it.

❖ **Moving your body is essential.** It is essential not only for weight loss, but for your overall health. Start out slow, don't push yourself. Take a walk with a friend or your poor dog that never gets out. As you lose weight, you will find that your energy level is higher and you will WANT TO EXERCISE. Really!

I never thought it could be true, but as I got thinner, I actually wanted to exercise because I had so much energy. It just feels so good for so many reasons! There are also lots of great online workout programs too if that's what turns you on. Keep it fun and interesting. I get my cardio exercise sometimes by turning up the music and dancing! Another benefit of exercise is that it is great for pivoting your thoughts. If you can't get out of a negative thought train, dance, run, jump to pivot your thoughts to healthy, positive ones that create the reality that you want!

❖ **Make your exercise count even more!** Another valuable use of your ability to choose your thoughts is to focus on the body part that you are exercising. I like to focus on the muscle that I am working and think about hard, lean muscles. It helps me to picture my muscles contracting and expanding and think about my body becoming stronger. Research says that you actually get more out of your movements that way.

❖ **Stay conscious when you eat**. If you are like me, you can go into a kind of food stupor and you don't even think or breath until everything on your plate is gone and then you wonder where it went! Put your fork down between every few bites, eat slowly, chew, chew, chew! I still have to remind myself to do this. It is a hard habit to break, but so important to do for your health and weight loss goals.

❖ **Once you get into a nice rhythm of eating healthy foods and exercise, do not focus on it anymore, just be, do, have it!** Use your focus instead of your new thin body that is coming. You don't want to be focusing on "losing weight" and "diets". The problem with focusing on losing weight is that you are feeding the vibration of "overweight" and "fat" which brings more opportunities to hang on to those things, through attracting yummy and fattening foods, more difficulty exercising, etc. By focusing, instead, on having a leaner body ... by finding places on your physical form that already please you and saying to the Universe, "I want more of this, please" ... you attract into your life new and fun ways to bring more leanness into your experience.

❖ **Be kind to yourself.** Don't beat yourself up if you fall off the health wagon and overeat. Just get right back on and continue. You deserve it and you are worth it. Congratulate yourself on the big and small victories and successes. I threw a party when I was able to cross my legs again with ease (but of course I didn't tell anyone what the party really was celebrating!)

❖ **Do not let yourself get to the starving point as that can lead to a major overeating binge.** It is always better to eat 6 small meals during the day, or at least have a snack between meals. I usually snack on nuts (don't go overboard, but they are a good source of protein and very filling) or fruits or both.

❖ **If you do end up in a binge**, do your best to still follow some rules such as, chewing slowly, putting your fork or spoon down between every several bites, breathing, staying conscious. Pull yourself out as soon as you can and do NOT bash yourself with negative talk. Just get right back on your program. Thin people overeat at times too. They just make up for it or continue with the way they were eating before.

❖ **About 'cheat days."** First of all, I would stop calling it cheating because that can lead to feelings of failure and a day of overeating is more likely to turn into a full-on binge and several days of overeating. If you really want something, like you are really obsessing about it, just eat it, following all rules of eating slowly, staying conscious, etc. and then get right back on the program. Don't make a big deal about it and don't set yourself up for a downward spiral. If you can stay conscious and just enjoy your food, you will be able to keep going without it turning into a day or weeks of overeating.

❖ **When you get into a plateau** and have not lost any weight for two weeks or more, I have a little secret, but you can only do this if you are very strong in your desire to keep losing weight. I have found that if I have a high calorie day of carbs, it tends to reset my body and I start losing weight again. You must be careful about this, because I know that when I am weak, a bowl of pasta can send me into a weeklong binge, but when I am strong, I can enjoy this day of reset and it gets my weight loss going again. Do not call it a "cheat day." This is a "reset day." And you must still follow all rules of eating slowly, chewing your food, staying conscious while you eat, etc.

❖ **Be very careful of the slippery slope of rewarding yourself with food.** It is best to reward yourself with new clothes, something you have been wanting, a day trip, or anything but food. Food is not your reward, a happy, healthy body is!

❖ **One of the best things you can do for your overall health and weight loss is to eat fresh, whole foods.** Fill your diet with whole foods like fruits, vegetables, nuts, seeds and whole grains. Foods that are still in their original, natural form. Highly processed breads, pastas, meats, sugar and other foods that no longer resemble what they once were will slow down your weight loss. Fried foods are out too, they are just horrible for your system. Become a lean, mean, greaseless machine! Widespread obesity and diabetes really are a thing of the last 30 to 40 years and it is directly related to highly processed foods and sugar.

❖ **You must get off the processed sugar.** It is doing all kinds of misdeeds with your body's chemical balance. Learn to love the sweetness and pure natural goodness of fruits. Natural Stevia is also an acceptable option. It might take a bit to end your cravings, but they will go away if you give your body a chance to adapt. It is worth it! You will feel so much better without the highs and big lows of too much sugar in your diet.

❖ **Give your body ten days without dairy and see what happens!** Dairy (milk) is for baby cows and there is a reason so many people have trouble processing it. Humans are the only species on Earth that continue to drink and use milk after weaning. You will find that a lot of your physical problems like lots of mucus, bloating, puffiness, indigestion and even moodiness plus so many other ills will magically go away once you get off dairy. If you are addicted to cheese, there are amazing vegan options in most stores now and fantastic recipes using cashews and other nuts and seeds that are very cheesy! However, as with everything do not go overboard and keep a caloric balance.

❖ **Explore Intermittent Fasting.** Many people report quick weight loss, improved health and studies show it may even help you live longer. Intermittent fasting is a way of eating that cycles between periods of fasting and eating. It does not specify which foods you should eat but rather when you should eat them. It is an eating pattern as opposed to a diet.

These are the most popular methods:

- **The 16/8 method:** This method involves restricting your daily eating period to 8 hours, such as 1:00 pm to 9 p.m. Then you fast for 16 hours in between. You can choose your hours according to your lifestyle. Usually, my eight hour eating period is from 9 am to 5 pm.

- **Eat-Stop-Eat:** This involves fasting for 24 hours, once or twice a week, for example by not eating from dinner one day until dinner the next day.

- **The 5:2 diet:** With this method, you consume only 500–600 calories on two non-consecutive days of the week but eat normally the other 5 days.

Intermittent fasting should not be mistaken for a food-free-for-all during your eating hours. If you shove in 3000 calories in those eight hours, it will not work for you. But if you are reasonable, you could find incredible results!

❖ **Practice control.** Unless you are really hungry, try waiting five minutes to eat and then five minutes more. Refer to your list of things to do instead of eating that you created earlier in this book.

❖ **You must be able to be okay with where you are.** It can get frustrating and you will be anxious because you are doing great, you are seeing the weight coming off, you are feeling good and you just want to be at your goal weight. Give your body a chance. Be okay with where you are and allow your success to spur you forward. If you are already looking in the mirror for a difference after starting a new diet only a few hours earlier, you must be patient!

❖ **Eating freestyle can be a slippery slope.** For me, it is best to be on a strict and laid out plan until I am really strong in my determination and motivation to lose weight. My favorite thing to do is to start out with a one day fast to really get myself mentally prepared. It is all downhill from there!

❖ **If you are going to sit and watch TV**, try sitting on a yoga ball so that you can keep moving while watching!

❖ **Decide if you want a quicker weight loss or a slower, but easier and steadier weight loss.** You can go on a stricter diet and lose weight faster or ease right into your new long term maintenance eating habits that will be permanent. This will cause a slower but more steady weight loss. Or you can do a combo of the two! You can do a stricter diet for three days of the week and a more maintenance diet the other four. It all depends on which feels best for you. You can also do one for a week and the other for the next week. Mix it up and go with your flow!

❖ **Find your caloric balance.** If you eat too few calories your body thinks you are starving and will hold onto that fat for dear life. And obviously if you eat too many calories, you will gain weight. And even when you find your balance that is working for you for a while, it can change. You have to be open to finding what works and not get frustrated as long as you are moving forward.

❖ **It is only food.** Use it to fortify your body and not fortify unhealthy food associations and patterns.

❖ **You are who you say you are.** So start singing out about how strong and amazing you are!

❖ **Do not let others determine your worth.** Only YOU and God can determine your worthiness and believe it, YOU ARE WORTHY!

❖ **Let others off the hook.** Get over people having to be a certain way to please you. You do you, Boo!

❖ **Be gentle with yourself.** It is not about focusing on what you have done wrong or mistakes you think you have made, as that just keeps you stuck there in self-pity and unworthiness. Yuck. Instead, focus on what you can and will do in this NOW moment to be fully and authentically who you already are; Love and Light Vibration. YES YOU ARE! *Retrain your brain to refrain from self-inflicted pain.* Change the tone of your self-talk to LOVE, GENTLENESS, PEACE, GRACE and EASE. Watch how worlds open up for you as you embrace the fine, divine being that YOU ARE. RIGHT NOW.

❖ **Do not eat when you are mad** or otherwise having negative thoughts as you do not want to literally feed your body this kind of energy. Get into a clear and balanced head space before you eat. Do not chew angrily.

- **When you get discouraged, remember how far you have come** and keep your eye on the prize. Remember where you are going and don't stay stuck on where you are.

- **Drink lots of water**. This helps with weight loss but will also help to keep your skin hydrated to avoid stretch marks and hanging skin. Use lots of lotion too!

- **Look in the mirror every day** and say "I Love You" and mean it, no matter where you are with your weight loss goals!

- **Get into the habit of saying thanks before you start your meal.** You do not have to be religious to give thanks to your food and anyone that helped to get it on your table including the farmers, truckers, store workers and especially God. This is part of being conscious about food and where it came from.

- **Know your patterns and food triggers**. I learned which situations caused me to overeat and I either avoided those situations or went with a plan. When I am really tired, my defenses are down and I tend to overeat. I also overeat if I let myself get too hungry and then I eat too much to make up for it. I tend to eat when I am bored and have nothing else to do, just out of habit. I made sure that I was busy doing the things that I love to do. I got myself inspired by my life again! When you are inspired, food is not so important, you have much better things to think about!

❖ **Don't allow yourself to feel deprived.** If you are hungry, truly hungry, EAT! I found it best to eat six smaller meals during the day than three big meals. Who made up the three meals a day rule anyway? It no longer made sense to me as I listened to my own body's guidance.

❖ **Do not skip meals.** I learned that it was important to keep my metabolism up and that skipping meals actually put my body into a starvation mode. I found out that your body starts to store fat instead of getting rid of it if it is not getting enough! I found a rhythm of eating and the kinds of foods that worked best for me. After time, I no longer followed the South Beach. I just ate the foods I enjoyed in reasonable amounts when I was hungry. I found some great raw snack bars and stocked up on those.

❖ **To weigh or not to weigh?** I went from alternatively weighing myself every day to every week and sometimes not for weeks. It just depended on what motivated and inspired me. I always followed my inner guidance. What motivated me the most was the way my clothes were getting bigger and bigger, and that is better than a number on a scale! The scale can be misleading, especially if you are exercising and developing muscle, which weighs more than fat. If I was not losing weight for a period of time, I would increase my tea/water consumption and exercise a little more.

❖ **Do not let cravings drive you crazy!** If I really wanted something, I ate it and then just got right back on the plan, just like thin people do. And if you are going to eat it, eat it with JOY! Guilt has a lot of calories! Then continue on with your plan without all the negative self-talk.

❖ **Plan what you are going to eat before going to the kitchen** instead of standing there with the refrigerator or cupboard door open. Have a plan and stick to it.

❖ **Allow yourself to be thin in your mind**, act like you already are, do the things you would do if you were thin. So many people put off their life "until I am thin" or "until I am rich" or "until I have that partner". All you have is NOW. Happiness and joy is a state that you need to feel right now, it is not "when I am thin" when I have money. For this to work, you need to feel that RIGHT NOW. How would you sit, how would you walk, how would you talk if you were thin? Do it NOW!

❖ **When you find an emotion that doesn't make you feel good, don't get mad** at yourself and beat yourself up about it, just fix it. Re-wire and refocus your thoughts. Say "I can change this now by changing my thoughts and perspective." Then Do it!

❖ **Let the mirror become your friend.** When I am not happy with myself and am not being all that I can be, I notice that I do not look in the mirror much, and when I do, I don't really see myself, I don't look myself in the eye. When I notice I am doing this, it is a sure sign that I need to work on raising my vibration/emotions/thoughts. I start doing the emotional work and I return to telling myself I love myself in the mirror!

❖ **Find a community of support.** Find like-minded friends, join my Webinars, Retreats, a community like our Becoming Thin Facebook Group or other similar communities. You do not have to and should not do this alone. Seek the support of others who will encourage you to listen to your own guidance (not just theirs!) and remind you to pivot your thoughts to always be thinking about that which you want!

AFFIRMATIONS

A ffirmations only work when you believe them, when you feel passionate about them, and allow yourself to feel the feelings of them already manifested. If you do not believe them at first, it's best to repeat them often and practice feeling how you would feel if the desire you are affirming for is already fulfilled. BE IT NOW!! FEEL IT NOW!!

It is beneficial to personalize affirmations so that they really resonate with YOU. The more you feel the affirmation is for YOU and about YOU, the faster you will see results. Affirmations are never written in stone, so continue to edit them to feel better or more focused on your outcome. It is common to edit your affirmations on a regular basis to keep them feeling fresh and evoking the emotions surrounding their anticipated outcome.

Be creative and really go for it! Affirm your desires, affirm your worthiness, and affirm your ideal body weight.

I believe that once you repeat affirmations several times over several days or several months, whatever it takes for you to truly believe them and feel passionate about them, you don't need to keep repeating them over and over. You will know when "it is done." I think that once you believe the affirmation and really feel it to be true, IT IS TRUE and you don't need to keep reaffirming over and over. You just let it go and let the Universe go to work! You do not have to keep asking. It is already done as soon as you believe it and know it to be true.

There are many affirmations listed here. You do not have to use all of them, in fact it would be quite overwhelming. Find the ones that feel good to you and resonate with you and copy those into your own journal. You can add new ones as it feels good!

Let us start off with my favorite affirmations that have created miracles for me. These were taught to me by my spiritual teacher, Marilyn, whom I mentioned at the beginning of the book. Write these down in your journal and see what happens!

The Divine Plan of my Life is manifesting for me now, quickly and in peace. Thank you, Thank you, Thank you!

The ___ (fill in the blank) I am seeking is seeking me and the Law of Good brings us together with love, ease and understanding. Thank you, Thank you, Thank you!

And now for the rest!

- I know that I can master anything, and I am in control of my life

- I Am going to relax and have fun with this, no matter what the outcome may be.

- I put my full trust in my inner guidance.

- I grow in strength with every forward step I take.

- I release my resistance now!

- I am making things easy for myself now.

- My body is getting stronger, slimmer, and healthier every day.

- I enjoy being healthy.

- I am on the road to fitness.

- I am thin.

- I am loving and lovable and I find love everywhere.

- I am enjoying how I am feeling now.

- I love the food that makes me healthy and thin.

- Losing weight is effortless.

- I am going to fit into the next size smaller any minute.

- I feel so thin inside, my outer is just about to catch up.

- It feels so good to have toned arms and legs.

- I create an abundance of energy when I work out.

- Exercise gives me a good feeling about myself.

- I will soon see results and that motivates me to get up every morning.

- My health is extremely important to me.

- Taking care of my body gives me great confidence.

- I am willing and committed to doing what it takes.

- I deserve healthy food and a healthy body.

- I will succeed at creating the body I have always wanted.

- I can see myself fitting into my smallest size clothes again.

- It will feel so nice to show off my body again.

- My body is to be kept beautiful, healthy, and sexy.

- I have fun and enjoy life when I am in good shape.

- Water satisfies my food cravings.

- I feel so good when I eat healthy.

- I enjoy wearing skinny clothes that show off my incredible body.

- Every time I exercise, I enjoy it more.

- Every day I notice positive changes in my mind and my body.

- I prefer to have a positive attitude.

- I am grateful for the ability to be active.

- I nurture myself by living a healthy lifestyle.

- As I strengthen my body, I strengthen my confidence and self-esteem.

- Getting in shape makes life so much easier.

- I am an inspiration to others.

- Getting in great shape is a worthy goal.

- The success I achieve in my health will rub off on the rest of my life.

- I am getting my whole life into balance.

- My body is my friend.

- I am never alone. The universe supports me and is with me at every step.

- My mind is filled only with loving, healthy, positive and prosperous thoughts which ultimately are converted into my life experiences.

- My mind is full of gratitude for my lovely and wonderful life.

- I consciously release the past and live only in the present. That way I get to enjoy and experience life to the full.

- Nothing tastes as good as thin feels.

- I send peaceful, loving thoughts to other people.

- I believe in myself.

- I love and accept my emotions.

- I am patient with myself.

- I am able to listen, understand and communicate openly and honestly with everyone I come in contact with.

- I appreciate myself. I give thanks for my wonderful life.

- I picture myself with a fit, trim and healthy body. As I picture it, I create it.

- I have the ability to feel the way I want at all times.

- I accept and love myself for who I am right now.

- My body is fit, healthy and strong.

- I listen to the wisdom of my heart.

- I laugh and play today.

- I give myself quiet time alone.

- I deserve to have a beautiful, fit and healthy body.

- I allow all good things to come to me.

- My days are filled with fun and meaningful activities.

- I bring love and a positive attitude to everything I do.

- I live my life to the fullest.

- I think about what is right and working in my life. I focus on the positive.

- I allow the gift of love to flow through me to others.

- I focus on what is good in people, thus assisting them in achieving it.

- I change the world around me by changing myself.

- My life is full of miracles.

- I am worthy of love and all good things.

- My dreams come true.

- I give thanks often. I appreciate all the beautiful things in my life.

- I trust that everything comes at the perfect time and in the perfect way.

- Every day I experience more love in my life.

- I give myself all that I need.

- I give myself permission to be happy.

- I am abundantly provided for as I follow my path.

- I follow my inner guidance.

- I focus on what is good and beautiful in my life. As I do, all that is good increases.

- I flow with the universe.

- All of my feelings are a part of myself and I love and accept all of my feelings.

- I listen within before taking action.

- I choose beliefs that bring me aliveness and growth.

- I love and honor everything I create.

- I forgive myself, knowing that I did the best I knew how at the time.

- I love getting there as much as being there.

- I smile and laugh often.

- I know my value. I honor my worth.

- I use all the energy around me to go higher.

- I follow my inner guidance over other peoples' advice.

- I love my body.

- I am my own best friend.

- I am balanced and centered at all times.

- Good things come to me easily.

- I follow my inner guidance to get things done easily and joyfully.

- I love and honor everything I create.

- I know what I love to do and I do it.

- My love raises the vibration of everything and everyone around me.

- My spiritual growth is a wonderful journey of discovery and adventure.

- I see the beauty in everything around me.

- I connect with the earth. I am grounded and centered.

- I see myself as growing and expanding.

- I appreciate all that I am and all that I have.

- I live in an abundant universe.

- I follow my highest joy.

- Whatever I give thanks for will increase.

- I follow my heart.

- I am that I am. And so it is.

- As I release anger and blame, my life becomes lighter, fuller and happier.

- All my experiences are opportunities to gain more power, clarity and vision.

- I speak highly of other people. I honor them with my words and thoughts.

- I am magnetic to my higher good and it is magnetic to me.

- I listen to the messages of my body.

- The things I create are even better than I imagine them to be.

- With each breath I increase the love in my life.

- I am love.

PRODUCTS AND SERVICES

There are some products and services that have really worked for me, and others that friends highly recommend. I invite you to use YOUR intuition and guidance to see if any of these things resonate with YOU. You can find more suggestions on my website at http://www.iam-iam-iam.com

The Land of I AM Store – features lots of I AM Affirmations on t-shirts, cups, picture frames and more! (http://www.cafepress.com/iamiamiam)

Torrid Clothing – was a Godsend to me while I was losing weight. Cute clothes at great prices (because your clothes won't fit you for long!)

EFT – Emotional Freedom Technique - EFT is a simple and powerful technique for clearing out blockages in the human subtle energy system by tapping on certain acupuncture points. The premise of EFT is that dis-ease – emotional or physical – is the result of a disruption or blockage in the energy field. When you clear out the blockage, health and wellbeing are easily restored. Anyone can learn the process, and EFT often works where nothing else will. EFT can help clear your energy system of the emotional roots of your weight gain and eating issues. This allows your body to normalize naturally, without struggle or deprivation. I will be providing videos and seminars on EFT for Weight Loss. Be sure you are on my mailing list to find out more. You can also visit http://www.eftuniverse.com/

Be sure you are on my **mailing list (**https://www.iam-iam-iam.com/contact-and-mailing-list/) for inspirational news, quotes and website, seminar, retreat and book updates.

www.ingramcontent.com/pod-product-compliance
Lightning Source LLC
Chambersburg PA
CBHW031411250726